21 Words
for Nurses

21 WORDS FOR NURSES

by Jeanine Young-Mason

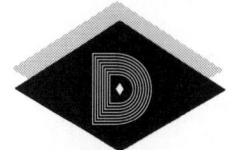

Diamond Communications, Inc.
South Bend, Indiana
1995

21 WORDS FOR NURSES

Copyright © 1995, by Jeanine Young-Mason

Manufactured in the
United States of America

Diamond Communications, Inc.
Post Office Box 88
South Bend, Indiana 46624
(219) 299-9278 • FAX (219) 299-9296
Orders: 800-480-3717

Library of Congress
Cataloging-in-Publication Data

Young-Mason, Jeanine, 1938-
    21 words for nurses / by Jeanine
    Young-Mason.
        p.   cm.
    Includes bibliographical references.
    ISBN 0-912083-85-9. --ISBN 0-912083-88-3
    1. Nursing--Philosophy--Quotations,
maxims, etc. 2. Nursing--Psychological
aspects--Quotations, maxims, etc. I. Title.
RT84.5.Y68   1995
610.73'01--dc20   95-30678
                                      CIP

To my sons,
Scott, Gregg, and Glenn.

CONTENTS

Introduction ix
Age 1
Anger 3
Balance 5
Change 7
Compassion 9
Discussion 11
Dislocation 13
Fear 15
Futility 17
Indifference 19
Illness 21
Knowledge 23
Meditation 25
Nursing 27
Perspective 29
Power 31
Self 33
Sorrow 35
Surviving 37
Understanding 39
World 41
Quotation Sources 43
Biosketch of Professor
    Jeanine Young-Mason 47

This little book of *21 WORDS FOR NURSES* highlights selected words which have particular relevance for nursing. They reflect ways of thinking about being and becoming a compassionate nurse. The quotations, offered as thoughts for meditation, are followed by enjoining comments. Additional space is provided for the reader to record personal reflections upon these words.

AGE

…there is wonder that only time can bestow. Age gives to all things, objects, institutions and individual lives, their value, their dignity, their worth. As a consequence, esteem should always turn upward to those who have gone ahead and stand before us.

Confucius

Nurses are intimate witnesses to the wonder and perplexities of age. Their esteem for the worth, the worthwhileness, of the wisdom of age invites others to share that reverence.

ANGER

I have learnt through bitter experience, one supreme lesson: to conserve my anger, and as heat conserved is transmuted into energy, even so our anger controlled can be transmuted into a power which can move the world.

Gandhi

There is much that angers the nurse who witnesses unnecessary suffering, disease, and death caused by arrogance, incompetence, indifference, and neglect. But when the force of that deep anger becomes disciplined intervention at all levels of the community, it has the potential to humanize every aspect of the health care system.

Balance

The caring component of nursing encompasses much more than a combination of the scientific and the technical. It encompasses and mandates a balance of the head, the heart, and the hands, or the science, the skill, and the spirit. We have forged ahead in the areas of science and technology, but there is fear among us that this spirit becomes dimmer and dimmer with the passage of time.

Isabella Stewart

Nurses have before them a unique opportunity today, and for the future, if nursing does not waver from what it has always known to be true; compassionate, humane care born out of deep reflection and desire is the antidote to institutionalized science and technology which has tilted health CARE toward an anonymous, sterile event.

CHANGE

There is nothing more difficult to carry out, nor more doubtful of success, nor more dangerous to handle, than to initiate a new order of things. For the reformer has enemies in all who profit by the old order of things, and only lukewarm defenders in all who profit by the new order. This luke-warmness arises partly from fear of their adversaries who have law in their favor, and partly from the incredulity of mankind who do not truly believe in anything new until they have had actual experience of it.

Niccolo Machiavelli

Before attempting to change the order of things for those you judge to be oppressed, however, take heed of your enthusiasm. Projects planned by outside agencies and change agents are often short sighted and sometimes their irresponsible actions have caused greater suffering. The intricate structures already in place may be necessary for survival.

COMPASSION

The act of compassion is costly. It makes us consciously aware of the agony around us, the spiritual and moral poverty.

Georges Bernanos

Compassion constitutes a radical form of criticism, for it announces that the hurt is to be taken seriously, that the hurt is not to be accepted as normal and natural, but it is an abnormal and unacceptable condition for humanness...Thus, compassion that might be seen simply as generous good will is, in fact, criticism of the system, forces, and ideologies that produce the hurt.

Walter Brueggemann

It should be clear that compassion is not mere sentimental emotion, nor is it an attempt to merely pity another. The compassionate act, thus defined, becomes the living basis for assisting those who are suffering. The complimentary ethics of compassion and advocacy may well be the most powerful, rewarding, and necessary acts of the nursing profession. Compassion, however, encompasses all those involved— physician, nurse, administrator, and clinician— in the care of the person, and no one exists above or beneath its power to make understanding possible and to heal.

DISCUSSION

We awoke them that they might question one another.

Koran

Discussion…stimulates the imagination and intellect by awakening the creative and inquisitive powers.

Mortimer Adler

Calm discussion provides the afflicted and the ill with the opportunity to respond fully, sharing their point of view, their values, their sense of what happened, what is happening, and what it means to them. In this honest and open atmosphere they, then, are able to exchange thought with the nurse and both can question one another, and both will be heard…and understood.

Dislocation

…the trauma of birth…the pathology of sickness…the morbidity of decrepitude …the phobia of death…to be tied to what one abhors…to be separated from what one loves…

Buddha

The constant anxiety engendered by being displaced from the source of life, comfort, health, facing hourly, daily, the abyss of the unknown or the detested known is dislocating of the human spirit.

FEAR

I have never caused anyone to weep. I have never spoken with a haughty voice. I have never made anyone afraid. I have never been deaf to words of justice and truth.

Egyptian Book of the Dead

Nursing might well adopt this ancient pledge, for in it is hidden a guide to compassionate nursing care.

FUTILITY

One of the greatest evils of the day…is a sense of futility. Young people say, 'What good can one person do? What is the sense of our small effort?' They cannot see that we must lay one brick at a time, take one step at a time: we can be responsible for only the one action of the present moment. But we can beg for an increase of love in our hearts that will vitalize and transform all our individual actions…

Dorothy Day

It is hard for many young nurses to imagine what influence one act of kindness, one compassionate intervention could accomplish in the life of another. But when a deep need is responded to, however brief the interaction, that person experiences a reprive from suffering. And, that reprive refreshes the spirit of both the sufferer and the nurse.

INDIFFERENCE

To many people, this indifference to truth or falsehood seems more comic than tragic. I find it tragic. It implies a frightful detachment, not only of the mind but of the entire person, even of the physical part of the person. Anyone who is indifferently open to truth or falsehood is ripe for any kind of tyranny. The passion for truth goes along with the passion for liberty. It is not for nothing that freedom of thought has always been regarded as the most precious of all freedoms, the one upon which all others depend.

Georges Bernanos

That "spiritual anemia" which is indifference has the potential to become a malignant condition. If unattended it develops into detachment and a paralyzing passivity in which the nurse surrenders rational judgement.

ILLNESS

Illness is the experience of living through the disease. If disease talk measures the body, illness talk tells of the fear and frustration of being inside a body that is breaking down. Illness begins where medicine leaves off, where I recognize that what is happening to my body happens to my life. My life consists of temperature and circulation, but also of hopes and disappointments, joys and sorrows, none of which can be measured. In illness talk there is no such thing as the body, only my body as I experience it. Disease talk charts the progression of certain measures. Illness talk is a story about moving from a perfectly comfortable body to one that forces me to ask: what's happening to me? Not it, but me.

Arthur Frank

Individuals cannot transcend "patient-hood" unless they are accepted as real with all of their difficulties and all of their sufferings—unless they are the reality and the illness is part of that reality. Any other perspective encourages dislocation of the human spirit, it is the antithesis of healing.

KNOWLEDGE

When you know a thing, to hold that you know it; and when you do not know a thing, to allow that you do not know it;— this is knowledge.

Confucius

The essential elements of knowledge for nursing means pursuing with thoroughness what is necessary to know and always being ready to recognize our limitations.

MEDITATION

Meditation is frequent and planned cogitation, which prudently investigates the cause and origin, the method and usefulness, of anything. Meditation has its beginning in reading, yet it is not constrained by any rules and precepts of reading. For it is delightful to have recourse to a certain suitable distance, where a free vision is possible for the contemplation of truth, and sometimes to touch lightly now these and then those causes of things, and sometimes to penetrate into them more deeply, and to leave nothing uncertain, and nothing obscure. The beginning of learning, therefore, is in reading, its consummation is in meditation. If anyone learns to love it intimately, and wants to have time for it more often, it bestows an exceedingly pleasant life, and offers the greatest consolation in time of trouble. For that is best which removes the spirit from the clash of earthly tumults, and also makes it possible in a certain sense to taste in this life the sweetness of everlasting peace.

Hugh of St. Victor

Meditation...no one can mandate it...it is utterly free...releasing the afflicted spirit of the nurse...enriching the mind.

Nursing

The real depths of nursing can only be made
  known
    through ideals,
    love,
    sympathy,
    knowledge,
    and culture,
    expressed through artistic practice.

Effie Taylor

A New art and a new science has been
created since and within the last forty years.
And with it a new profession—so they say;
we say, *calling*…the art of *nursing the sick*.
Please mark…*nursing the sick*; NOT nursing
the sickness…(what is health nursing?)… the
cultivation of health…What is Sickness?…
Nature's way of getting rid of the effects of
conditions which have interfered with health.
It is nature's attempt to cure. We have to help
her…What is health? Health is not only to be
well, but to use well every power we
have…What is nursing? Both kinds of nursing are to put us in the best possible conditions
for Nature to restore or preserve health…We
are only on the threshold of nursing.

Florence Nightingale

PERSPECTIVE

There was something else, something indescribable but as real as dim colour or soft sound. It was the spirit of the place: the countryside was faintly magical even in the rain. Half-tones told of it: and the soft atmosphere made you feel that you were in a region that was your proper home, a home where there was neither time, nor tide, nor any change at all, something friendly and akin and full of all that might be needed, if need were to arise; but it never did, for you felt that nothing was lacking. And you did not want to speak.

Oliver St. John Gogarty

The magical transformation of perspective found in nature is crucial for those in need of healing in the world of the clinic, hospital, doctor's office, and nursing home. The bleakness and often cruelly sterile atmosphere diminishes caregivers and sufferers alike and often thwarts healing. Artists (such as Gogarty) in every culture and throughout history have sought inspiration from nature, and by their own experience in their art, they have evoked for others the human need to rediscover and be re-juvenated by its kindredness and its plenitude.

POWER

All of us dwell on the brink of the infinite ocean of life's creative power. We all carry it within us; supreme strength, the fullness of wisdom, unquenchable joy. It is never thwarted and cannot be destroyed. But it is hidden deep, which is what makes life a problem. The infinite is down in the darkest, profoundest vault of our being, in the forgotten well-house, the deep cistern. What if we could discover it again and draw from it unceasingly?

Huston Smith

How can the nurse discover this hidden, powerful self? Through desire and devotion to reading, reflection, the perspective of nature, the enlightenment of meaningful conversation, through deep friendship, through knowledge, through the experience of compassion.

SELF

You are your thoughts, brother,
   the rest of you is bones and fiber,
If you think of roses,
      you are a rosegarden,
   but if you think of thorns,
      you are fire's fuel.

Rumi

The nurse's devotion to the ideal ethics of advocacy and compassion requires the disciplined development of a personal philosophy which, then, infuses every thought and every action, which then constitutes the nurse.

Sorrow

                    Why? Why did they
Have to die! I couldn't understand. I asked
Unanswerable questions a child asks
When a parent dies—for nothing. Only slowly
Did I make myself believe—or hope—they
Might all be swept up in their fragments
Together
And made whole again
By some compassionate hand.
But my hand was too small
To do the gathering.
I have only known this feeling since
When I look out across the sea of death,
This pull inside against a littleness—myself—
Waiting for an upward gesture.

> *Herbert Mason, a retelling*
> *of* Gilgamesh

Nurses endure the sorrow of loss in great
measure and they are humbled and mystified by
its magnitude. Their indomitable desire to make
lives whole again is kindled by a deep yearning
for the "upward gesture" of hope for all.

SURVIVING

Survive, is that the word for it
for what one does
for what one is

One's enemies abound
with truths and partial truths
that want to kill
before one can embrace
the truth one yearns to hold

The volunteers for truth abound
the esoteric squad
one knows if one has truly lived

They fear that imperfection
may reflect on them
if it is overlooked
and left to grow
and mar the definition
they have given life

Survive, for what?
to be content to live with hope
not bitterness:
survive to lose oneself
for other reasons
than the flaws
one knows exist

Surviving *by Herbert Mason*

We don't live only to survive but to aspire to
our fullest human and spiritual capacities.

UNDERSTANDING

For in the final analysis, we feel and understand only the tips of things presented to us in this world that are able to impress our senses and our soul. But everything else continues into infinite darkness. And even though they are close at hand, a thousand things are hidden because we are not capable of grasping them.

Auguste Rodin

Nurses must recognize that everything is truly close at hand and yet at the same time mysterious and elusive as life itself that is in their care.

WORLD

For the world is not atoms or molecules or radio-activity or other forces, the diamond is not carbon, and light is not vibrations of ether. You can never come to the reality of creation by contemplating it from the point of view of destruction.

Tagore

The world to the nurse is there to see, to know, to revere most positively in its plenitude; and each person is the life of that seeing and knowing and that plenitude.

QUOTATION SOURCES

Adler, Mortimer. *The Paideia Proposal.*
Collier Books, McMillan: New York,
1982, p. 29.

Bernanos, Georges. "Why Freedom?"
The Last Essays of George Bernanos. Trans. by
Joan & Barry Ulanov, Henry Regenery:
Chicago, 1955, p. 117.

Brueggemann, Walter. *Prophetic Imagination.*
Fortress Press: Philadelphia, 1978,
p. 85, 86.

Buddha in *Religions of Man.* Huston Smith.
Harper & Row: New York, 1986,
p. 151, 152.

Confucius in *Portable World Bible.* Ed. by
Robert O. Ballou.
Penguin: Harmondsworth,
1972, p.500.

Day, Dorothy. *Loaves and Fishes.*
Haper & Row: New York, 1983.

Egyptian *Book of the Dead* in *Waiting for God.*
Simone Weil. Harper & Row: New York,
1951, p.144.

Frank, Arthur. *At the Will of the Body:
Reflections on Illness.* Houghton Miflin:
Boston, 1991, p. 13.

Gandhi in *The Words of Gandhi.* Ed. by
Richard Attenborough. New Mark Press:
New York, 1982, p.13.

21 Words for Nurses

St. John Gogarty in "The Spirit of the Place" in "Nursing and the Arts" *Clinical Nurse Specialist.* Jeanine Young-Mason. (1993) vol. 7 (6), p. 318.

Hugh of St. Victor. "On Study and Teaching" *The Portable Medieval Reader.* Ed. by James Bruce Ross and Mary Martin McLaughlin. Penguin: New York, 1977, p. 581.

Koran. Tr. M.M. Pickthal. Mentor: New York. 9th printing, 1953, 18:20.

Machiavelli, Niccolo. *The Prince.* Penguin: Harmondsworth, 1970.

Mason, Herbert. *Gilgamesh,* a retelling. Mentor NAL: New York, 1972, p. 78, 79.

Mason, Herbert, "Surviving" *Sufi,* London. vol. 25, 1995.

Nightingale, Florence. "Sick Nursing and Health Nursing" in *Woman's Mission,* Burdett Coutts. London, 1893, p. 184-86, 198.

Rumi, *Mathnawi,* ed. R.A. Nicholson (1925-1940), Book II, V. 277-278.

Rodin, Auguste. *Art: Conversations with Paul Gsell.* Trans. by deCaso, J. & P.B. Sanders. University of California Press: Berkeley. 1984, p. 82.

QUOTATION SOURCES

Smith, Huston. *Religions of Man.*
Harper & Row: New York. 1986, p. 43.

Stewart, Isabella. "The Science and the Art
of Nursing." (Editorial) *Nursing
Education Bulletin.* 1929, 2:1.

Tagore, Rabindranath. *Upanishads.* Ed. by
Juan Mascaro. Penguin: New York,
1971, p. 17.

Taylor, Effie. "Of What is the Nature
of Nursing?" *American Journal of Nursing.*
(1934) Vol. 34.

BIOSKETCH OF PROFESSOR JEANINE YOUNG-MASON

Jeanine Young-Mason, Ed. D., R.N., C.S., F.A.A.N., is Associate Professor of Nursing at the University of Massachusetts at Amherst where she teaches writing seminars in nursing studies and community health nursing and consultation in the graduate and undergraduate programs. She is a psychiatric-mental health clinical nurse specialist with a Doctorate in Humanistic and Behavioral Studies from Boston University. Young-Mason's writing, research, teaching, and consultation center on literature and the arts as primary sources for the study of suffering and compassion. She is specifically interested in the way in which nurses are educated to approach human suffering—pragmatically, morally, and spiritually. Young-Mason writes a regular column on "Nursing and the Arts" in *Clinical Nurse Specialist*. She is the author of *States of Exhile: Correspondences Between Art and Literature and Nursing Phenomena* (NLN Press, NYC, June 1995) and the forthcoming *Chronicles of the Ill* (F.A. Davis, Philadelphia, Spring 1996).